Copyright © 2023 by Herman Strange (Author)

All rights reserved. This book or any portion thereof may not be reproduced or used in any manner whatsoever without the express written permission of the publisher except for the use of brief quotations in a book review.

This book is copyright protected. This is only for personal use. You cannot amend, distributor, sell, use, quote or paraphrase any part or the content within this book without the consent of the author. Please note the information contained within this document is for educational and entertainment purposes only. Every attempt has been made to provide accurate, up to date and reliable complete information. No warranties of any kind are expressed or implied.

Readers acknowledge that the author is not engaging in the rendering of legal, financial, medical or professional advice. The content of this book has been derived from various sources. Please consult a licensed professional before attempting any techniques outlined in this book.

By reading this document, the readers agree that under no circumstances are the author responsible for any losses, direct or indirect, which are incurred as a result of the use of information contained within this document, including but not limited to errors, omissions or inaccuracies.

Thank you very much for reading this book.

Title: Check-Ups for Health-Understanding the Importance of Preventive Care
Subtitle: A Guide to Essential Health Screenings and Preventive Measures

Series: Healthy Habits for Life: Building Sustainable Habits for Optimal Health and Wellness
Author: Serenity Tanner

Table of Contents

Introduction 5
Understanding the Need for Preventive Care 5
Overcoming Barriers to Preventive Care 8

Chapter 1: The Basics of Regular Medical Check-Ups 12
The importance of preventive care 12
Understanding the types of medical exams 14
How often should you get a check-up? 16

Chapter 2: Physical Exams and Screening Tests 18
The role of physical exams in early detection and prevention of disease 18
The benefits of common screening tests, such as blood pressure and cholesterol checks 21
Understanding the importance of cancer screenings 24

Chapter 3: Mental Health Screenings 26
The benefits of regular mental health screenings 26
Understanding common mental health conditions 29
How to identify signs and symptoms of mental health issues 32

Chapter 4: Understanding Medical Reports and Test Results 35
Interpreting medical reports and lab test results 35

How to communicate effectively with healthcare providers 39

Understanding medical jargon 42

Chapter 5: Special Considerations for Different Age Groups 45

Age-appropriate health screenings 45

Understanding common health risks for different age groups 49

Preventive care for children, adults, and seniors 53

Chapter 6: Overcoming Barriers to Regular Check-Ups 57

Financial and insurance barriers to care 57

Overcoming fear and anxiety about medical exams 62

The role of patient education in preventive care 64

Conclusion" 67

The Importance of Taking Action 67

Looking Towards the Future 69

Potential References 71

Introduction

Understanding the Need for Preventive Care

Taking care of your health is one of the most important things you can do for yourself. Your body is a complex machine that requires proper care and maintenance to function at its best. While there are many things you can do to promote good health, one of the most important is to engage in preventive care.

Preventive care refers to a range of medical services that are designed to help you stay healthy and prevent illness before it occurs. This type of care includes regular check-ups, screenings, and tests that can help detect health problems early on, when they are most treatable. By engaging in preventive care, you can help reduce your risk of developing chronic conditions, such as diabetes, heart disease, and cancer, and improve your overall health and well-being.

The Importance of Preventive Care

Preventive care is important for several reasons. First, it can help detect health problems early on, before they have a chance to develop into more serious conditions. For example, regular cancer screenings can help detect cancer in its early stages, when it is most treatable. Similarly, routine blood pressure and cholesterol checks can help detect the early signs of heart disease, which can be managed with lifestyle changes and medications.

Second, preventive care can help you manage existing health conditions. For example, if you have diabetes, regular check-ups with your healthcare provider can help you monitor your blood sugar levels and make necessary adjustments to your treatment plan. By managing your condition proactively, you can help prevent complications and improve your quality of life.

Third, engaging in preventive care can help you establish a positive relationship with your healthcare provider. Regular check-ups provide an opportunity for you to discuss any health concerns you may have and ask questions about your health. This can help you feel more informed and empowered to take an active role in managing your health.

The Benefits of Preventive Care

Engaging in preventive care has many benefits, including:

- Improved health outcomes: By detecting and managing health problems early on, you can help prevent complications and improve your overall health outcomes.

- Cost savings: Preventive care can help you avoid more expensive treatments and hospitalizations down the line.

- Better quality of life: By managing existing health conditions and preventing new ones, you can improve your quality of life and reduce the impact of illness on your daily activities.

- Peace of mind: Knowing that you are taking proactive steps to manage your health can provide peace of mind and reduce anxiety about potential health problems.

In summary, preventive care is an important aspect of maintaining good health. By engaging in regular check-ups, screenings, and tests, you can help detect health problems early on, manage existing conditions, and improve your overall health and well-being.

Overcoming Barriers to Preventive Care

Preventive care is an essential aspect of maintaining good health, but many individuals face barriers that prevent them from receiving regular check-ups and screenings. Some of the common barriers include financial constraints, lack of access to healthcare, and fear or anxiety about medical exams. This section will explore these barriers in more detail and provide strategies for overcoming them.

Financial Barriers

One of the most significant barriers to preventive care is financial constraints. Many people cannot afford to pay for regular medical exams and screenings out of pocket, and even those with insurance may face high deductibles and co-payments. As a result, they may avoid seeking preventive care altogether, putting their health at risk.

Fortunately, there are several strategies for overcoming financial barriers to preventive care. One option is to look for free or low-cost clinics in your area that offer preventive care services. Many community health centers offer discounted services based on income and can provide basic preventive care, such as blood pressure and cholesterol checks, immunizations, and cancer screenings.

Another option is to take advantage of preventive care services covered by insurance plans. Under the Affordable

Care Act, many insurance plans are required to cover certain preventive services, such as mammograms, colonoscopies, and flu shots, without cost-sharing. It is essential to understand what preventive services are covered by your insurance plan and take advantage of them.

Lack of Access to Healthcare

Another significant barrier to preventive care is a lack of access to healthcare. This may be due to living in a rural area without access to healthcare facilities, lack of transportation to healthcare facilities, or a shortage of healthcare providers in your area.

One way to overcome this barrier is to use telemedicine services. Telemedicine allows patients to connect with healthcare providers through video conferencing, phone calls, or messaging. This can be particularly helpful for individuals who live in remote areas or have difficulty traveling to healthcare facilities.

Another option is to take advantage of mobile healthcare services. Many healthcare providers offer mobile services, such as health screenings and check-ups, that can be brought directly to your community or workplace.

Fear and Anxiety about Medical Exams

Fear and anxiety about medical exams are common barriers to preventive care. Some individuals may avoid check-ups and screenings due to a fear of receiving bad news or being diagnosed with a serious illness. Others may have had negative experiences with healthcare providers in the past and are reluctant to seek care.

One way to overcome this barrier is to find a healthcare provider who puts you at ease. This may involve finding a provider who listens to your concerns and takes the time to explain procedures and test results in a way that you can understand. It may also involve finding a provider who offers a comfortable and welcoming environment.

Another strategy for overcoming fear and anxiety about medical exams is to educate yourself about the importance of preventive care and the benefits of regular check-ups and screenings. Understanding how preventive care can help you maintain good health and prevent serious illnesses can help alleviate some of the anxiety associated with medical exams.

Conclusion

In conclusion, preventive care is an essential aspect of maintaining good health, but many individuals face barriers that prevent them from receiving regular check-ups and screenings. By understanding and overcoming these barriers, individuals can take control of their health and improve their overall well-being. Strategies such as taking advantage of free or low-cost clinics, using telemedicine services, and finding a healthcare provider who puts you at ease can help individuals overcome financial, access, and anxiety barriers to preventive care.

Chapter 1: The Basics of Regular Medical Check-Ups

The importance of preventive care

Preventive care is essential for maintaining good health and preventing diseases. It involves taking proactive steps to identify and address health issues before they become serious or life-threatening. Preventive care can include regular check-ups, screening tests, vaccinations, and lifestyle changes.

Preventive care is important for several reasons. First, it can help detect diseases early, when they are most treatable. Many diseases, such as cancer and heart disease, are easier to treat and have better outcomes when detected in their early stages. Second, preventive care can help reduce healthcare costs by preventing the need for more expensive treatments and hospitalizations. Third, preventive care can improve quality of life by reducing the impact of chronic conditions and preventing complications.

Regular medical check-ups are a critical component of preventive care. During a check-up, your healthcare provider can assess your overall health, identify risk factors, and recommend appropriate screening tests and lifestyle changes. By detecting potential health problems early, you and your healthcare provider can work together to address them before they become serious.

In addition to regular check-ups, there are other preventive measures you can take to maintain good health. For example, following a healthy diet, getting regular exercise, and avoiding tobacco and excessive alcohol consumption can all reduce your risk of developing chronic conditions such as diabetes, heart disease, and certain types of cancer. Vaccinations are also an important part of preventive care, as they can protect you from serious infectious diseases such as influenza and hepatitis.

Overall, the importance of preventive care cannot be overstated. By taking proactive steps to maintain your health, you can reduce your risk of developing serious health conditions, improve your quality of life, and save money on healthcare costs. If you haven't already, schedule a check-up with your healthcare provider today to start taking control of your health.

Understanding the types of medical exams

Medical exams are a critical component of preventive care. They can help detect potential health problems early, when they are most treatable, and allow healthcare providers to develop personalized recommendations to help you maintain good health. Here are some of the most common types of medical exams:

1. Physical Exams: A physical exam is a comprehensive evaluation of your overall health. During a physical exam, your healthcare provider will typically take your medical history, check your vital signs (such as blood pressure and heart rate), and examine your body from head to toe for signs of potential health problems.

2. Diagnostic Tests: Diagnostic tests are used to identify potential health problems or to confirm a diagnosis. Common diagnostic tests include blood tests, urine tests, and imaging tests such as X-rays and MRIs.

3. Screening Tests: Screening tests are used to detect potential health problems before symptoms appear. These tests are typically recommended based on age, gender, and other risk factors. Common screening tests include mammograms, Pap smears, and colonoscopies.

4. Immunizations: Immunizations, or vaccines, are used to protect against infectious diseases such as influenza,

hepatitis, and HPV. Immunizations are typically recommended based on age and other risk factors.

5. Specialized Exams: Depending on your medical history and risk factors, your healthcare provider may recommend specialized exams such as vision and hearing tests, skin exams, or mental health screenings.

It's important to understand the types of medical exams that are appropriate for your age, gender, and medical history. Your healthcare provider can help you develop a personalized plan for preventive care that includes the appropriate types of exams and tests.

In addition to understanding the types of medical exams, it's also important to know how often you should be getting these exams. The frequency of medical exams can vary based on your age, medical history, and other risk factors. Your healthcare provider can help you determine how often you should be getting regular check-ups and other medical exams.

Overall, understanding the types of medical exams is an important part of taking control of your health. By working with your healthcare provider to develop a personalized plan for preventive care, you can detect potential health problems early and maintain good health for years to come.

How often should you get a check-up?

Regular medical check-ups are an essential part of preventive care. But how often should you get a check-up? The answer depends on several factors, such as age, gender, overall health status, and family medical history.

For children and adolescents, regular check-ups are critical for monitoring their growth and development. Pediatricians typically recommend annual check-ups for children and adolescents to assess their physical, emotional, and social well-being. During these visits, healthcare providers may also administer vaccines, conduct vision and hearing tests, and screen for common health issues such as obesity and mental health conditions.

For adults, the frequency of check-ups may vary depending on their health status and risk factors. Generally, adults should get a check-up at least once a year. However, certain populations, such as those with chronic conditions like diabetes or heart disease, may need to see their healthcare provider more frequently. Women may also require additional screenings and exams, such as mammograms and pap tests.

It's important to note that even if you feel healthy, you should still get regular check-ups. Many health conditions, such as high blood pressure and high cholesterol, often have no noticeable symptoms. Regular check-ups can help detect these conditions early, when they are more treatable.

Other factors that may influence how often you should get a check-up include your family medical history, lifestyle habits, and occupation. For example, if you have a family history of cancer or heart disease, you may need to get screened more frequently. Similarly, if you work in a high-risk occupation, such as construction or healthcare, you may need more frequent screenings for occupational hazards.

In conclusion, the frequency of medical check-ups depends on various factors, including age, gender, health status, and risk factors. While annual check-ups are generally recommended for adults, certain populations may need to see their healthcare provider more frequently. Ultimately, the best way to determine how often you should get a check-up is to consult with your healthcare provider and develop a personalized preventive care plan.

Chapter 2: Physical Exams and Screening Tests
The role of physical exams in early detection and prevention of disease

Physical exams are an essential component of preventive healthcare, as they provide an opportunity for healthcare providers to identify potential health problems before they become severe. Physical exams involve a thorough evaluation of the body's systems, including the cardiovascular, respiratory, neurological, and musculoskeletal systems, among others. During a physical exam, a healthcare provider may also perform various screening tests to detect early signs of diseases, such as cancer or heart disease.

Early detection of diseases through physical exams and screening tests can be crucial in preventing severe health consequences. For example, mammograms and colonoscopies are common screening tests that can detect breast and colon cancers in their early stages, when they are more treatable. Similarly, blood pressure checks and cholesterol screenings can detect cardiovascular disease before it becomes life-threatening.

Physical exams are particularly important for individuals with a family history of specific diseases or conditions, as they may be at a higher risk for developing those conditions. For example, if someone's family has a history of diabetes, their healthcare provider may perform regular blood sugar screenings to detect early signs of the disease.

In addition to detecting potential health problems, physical exams also serve as an opportunity for healthcare providers to educate patients about healthy lifestyle choices. During a physical exam, a healthcare provider may discuss topics such as nutrition, exercise, and stress management, as well as provide advice on how to make healthier choices to improve overall health and reduce the risk of developing certain conditions.

It is also essential to note that physical exams are not a one-time event but should be performed regularly, depending on an individual's age, gender, and medical history. For example, individuals between the ages of 20 and 40 may only require physical exams every few years, while individuals over the age of 40 may require yearly exams.

In conclusion, physical exams play a crucial role in the early detection and prevention of diseases. They provide an opportunity for healthcare providers to identify potential health problems before they become severe, as well as an opportunity to educate patients on healthy lifestyle choices. Regular physical exams are essential, and individuals should work with their healthcare providers to determine the appropriate frequency of exams based on their age, gender, and medical history. By prioritizing regular physical exams, individuals can take control of their health and prevent potential health problems before they become severe.

The benefits of common screening tests, such as blood pressure and cholesterol checks

Regular screening tests are an essential part of preventive care as they help detect early signs of disease and enable early intervention. Two of the most common screening tests are blood pressure and cholesterol checks. These tests are simple, inexpensive, and can be done during a regular check-up.

Blood Pressure Screening:

High blood pressure or hypertension is a silent killer that can lead to heart attacks, strokes, and kidney damage. According to the American Heart Association, more than 100 million adults in the United States have high blood pressure, and only about half have it under control.

A blood pressure screening test involves measuring the pressure of the blood against the walls of the arteries. The test is usually performed using a sphygmomanometer, which consists of an inflatable cuff and a pressure gauge. The test is painless and takes only a few minutes.

The results of a blood pressure test are expressed as two numbers: systolic pressure (the pressure when the heart beats) and diastolic pressure (the pressure when the heart rests between beats). A normal blood pressure reading is less than 120/80 mmHg. If the reading is between 120/80 and

139/89 mmHg, it is considered prehypertension, and lifestyle changes may be recommended to prevent the development of high blood pressure. If the reading is 140/90 mmHg or higher, it is considered high blood pressure, and medical intervention may be required.

The Benefits of Blood Pressure Screening:

Blood pressure screening is a crucial tool for preventing heart attacks, strokes, and kidney damage. By detecting high blood pressure early, lifestyle changes and medications can be prescribed to reduce blood pressure and lower the risk of complications.

Cholesterol Screening:

Cholesterol is a type of fat that is essential for the body's functioning. However, high levels of cholesterol in the blood can lead to the buildup of plaque in the arteries, increasing the risk of heart disease and stroke.

A cholesterol screening test involves measuring the levels of total cholesterol, LDL (bad) cholesterol, HDL (good) cholesterol, and triglycerides in the blood. The test is usually performed after a period of fasting, as eating can affect cholesterol levels. The test is painless and takes only a few minutes.

The results of a cholesterol test are expressed as the levels of the different types of cholesterol and triglycerides. A normal cholesterol level is less than 200 mg/dL. If the level of LDL cholesterol is high, lifestyle changes and medications may be recommended to reduce the risk of heart disease and stroke.

The Benefits of Cholesterol Screening:

Cholesterol screening is a crucial tool for preventing heart disease and stroke. By detecting high cholesterol levels early, lifestyle changes and medications can be prescribed to reduce cholesterol levels and lower the risk of complications.

In conclusion, regular screening tests such as blood pressure and cholesterol checks are essential tools for preventive care. They can help detect early signs of disease and enable early intervention, reducing the risk of complications and improving health outcomes. It is recommended to discuss screening tests with a healthcare provider to determine the appropriate frequency and type of tests based on individual risk factors and medical history.

Understanding the importance of cancer screenings

Cancer is a serious disease that affects millions of people around the world every year. The earlier cancer is detected, the better the chances of successful treatment and recovery. This is why cancer screening is so important, and why it is a critical part of regular medical check-ups.

Cancer screening is a process that involves testing for the presence of cancer before any symptoms appear. This can be done using a variety of tests, depending on the type of cancer being screened for. Some of the most common cancer screening tests include mammograms for breast cancer, colonoscopies for colon cancer, and pap smears for cervical cancer.

There are many benefits to cancer screening. Perhaps the most important benefit is early detection. When cancer is caught early, it is much easier to treat and the chances of successful treatment are much higher. In some cases, early detection can even lead to a complete cure. Cancer screening can also help identify people who are at high risk for developing certain types of cancer, so that they can take steps to reduce their risk.

Despite the benefits of cancer screening, some people may be hesitant to undergo these tests. One reason for this is fear or anxiety about the test itself or the possibility of a cancer diagnosis. It is important to remember, however, that early detection is key to successful treatment, and that many types of cancer can be treated successfully if caught early.

Another barrier to cancer screening is the cost. Some screening tests can be expensive, and not all insurance plans cover them. However, many healthcare providers offer free or low-cost cancer screening programs, and some programs even offer financial assistance to help cover the cost of screening.

It is important to talk to your healthcare provider about your individual risk factors for cancer and to discuss which screening tests are right for you. By understanding the importance of cancer screening and taking steps to overcome barriers to screening, you can take an active role in maintaining your health and reducing your risk of cancer.

Chapter 3: Mental Health Screenings

The benefits of regular mental health screenings

Mental health is a crucial aspect of overall well-being, and just like physical health, it requires regular attention and care. Mental health screenings are an important tool in identifying and addressing potential mental health issues early on, before they develop into more serious problems. In this section, we'll discuss the benefits of regular mental health screenings and why they should be a part of everyone's preventive care routine.

1. Early Detection and Treatment

One of the most significant benefits of regular mental health screenings is early detection and treatment. Just like with physical health conditions, early detection of mental health problems can make a significant difference in treatment outcomes. By catching mental health issues early, individuals can seek appropriate treatment and support, which can help prevent symptoms from becoming more severe or chronic.

2. Improved Quality of Life

Regular mental health screenings can also improve an individual's overall quality of life. When mental health conditions go untreated, they can have a significant impact on an individual's daily functioning, relationships, and ability to participate in activities they enjoy. By identifying and treating mental health issues early, individuals can get the support they need to manage their symptoms and improve their quality of life.

3. Reduced Stigma

Another benefit of regular mental health screenings is reducing the stigma associated with mental health issues. By making mental health a routine part of preventive care, individuals can help reduce the shame and embarrassment that many people feel about seeking mental health treatment. Regular screenings can also help normalize discussions around mental health and encourage individuals to seek help when they need it.

4. Increased Awareness and Understanding

Regular mental health screenings can also increase an individual's awareness and understanding of mental health issues. By taking the time to assess their mental health regularly, individuals can become more familiar with the signs and symptoms of common mental health conditions. This increased awareness can help individuals recognize potential mental health issues in themselves and others and encourage them to seek support.

5. Improved Mental Health Literacy

Finally, regular mental health screenings can improve an individual's mental health literacy. Mental health literacy refers to the knowledge and understanding of mental health conditions, treatment options, and available resources. By participating in regular mental health screenings, individuals can learn more about mental health and become better equipped to manage their own mental health needs.

In conclusion, regular mental health screenings are a valuable tool for maintaining overall well-being and preventing mental health issues from becoming more severe. By detecting and treating mental health problems early, individuals can improve their quality of life and reduce the stigma associated with mental health issues. Regular screenings can also increase awareness and understanding of mental health issues, improving mental health literacy and encouraging individuals to seek help when they need it.

Understanding common mental health conditions

Mental health conditions are common and can affect anyone, regardless of age, gender, or background. These conditions can be caused by a variety of factors, including genetic predisposition, environmental factors, and life experiences. In this chapter, we will discuss some of the most common mental health conditions that people may experience.

1. Anxiety Disorders Anxiety disorders are a group of conditions characterized by excessive worry, fear, or panic. Some common types of anxiety disorders include generalized anxiety disorder, panic disorder, and social anxiety disorder. Symptoms may include feelings of nervousness, restlessness, difficulty concentrating, and physical symptoms such as sweating, trembling, and shortness of breath. Treatment options for anxiety disorders may include therapy, medication, or a combination of both.

2. Mood Disorders Mood disorders are a group of conditions that affect a person's emotional state. Some common types of mood disorders include major depressive disorder and bipolar disorder. Symptoms of these conditions may include feelings of sadness, hopelessness, or emptiness, as well as changes in sleep patterns, appetite, and energy

levels. Treatment for mood disorders may involve therapy, medication, or a combination of both.

3. Eating Disorders Eating disorders are a group of conditions characterized by abnormal eating habits that may negatively impact a person's physical and mental health. Some common types of eating disorders include anorexia nervosa, bulimia nervosa, and binge-eating disorder. Symptoms may include restricting food intake, purging behaviors, or episodes of binge eating. Treatment for eating disorders may involve therapy, medication, and nutritional counseling.

4. Substance Use Disorders Substance use disorders are a group of conditions characterized by the problematic use of drugs or alcohol. These conditions can lead to physical and mental health problems, as well as social and legal consequences. Treatment options for substance use disorders may include therapy, medication-assisted treatment, and support groups.

5. Personality Disorders Personality disorders are a group of conditions characterized by persistent patterns of behavior, thoughts, and feelings that deviate from societal norms. Some common types of personality disorders include borderline personality disorder, narcissistic personality disorder, and antisocial personality disorder. Symptoms may

include unstable relationships, impulsivity, and difficulty regulating emotions. Treatment options for personality disorders may include therapy, medication, and support groups.

In conclusion, mental health conditions are common and can affect anyone. By understanding the signs and symptoms of these conditions, individuals can seek treatment and support to improve their mental health and overall well-being.

How to identify signs and symptoms of mental health issues

Mental health issues can be difficult to identify and even harder to talk about. However, early identification and treatment of these conditions can significantly improve a person's quality of life. Here are some tips on how to identify signs and symptoms of mental health issues:

1. Know the common signs and symptoms of mental health issues: Mental health issues can manifest in a variety of ways, and it's important to recognize the signs and symptoms. Common signs include changes in mood, behavior, or thinking patterns, increased irritability or agitation, withdrawal from social activities or relationships, changes in appetite or sleep patterns, and difficulty concentrating or making decisions.

2. Pay attention to physical symptoms: Mental health issues can also have physical symptoms, such as chronic pain, headaches, digestive problems, or fatigue. These physical symptoms may be a sign of an underlying mental health issue.

3. Monitor changes in behavior: It's important to pay attention to changes in behavior, such as sudden mood swings, reckless behavior, or increased use of drugs or

alcohol. These changes may indicate an underlying mental health issue.

4. Talk to loved ones: If you notice changes in behavior or mood, it's important to talk to your loved ones about your concerns. They may be able to provide additional insights or help you identify patterns that you might not have noticed.

5. Seek professional help: If you or a loved one is experiencing symptoms of mental health issues, it's important to seek professional help. Mental health professionals, such as therapists or psychiatrists, can provide a diagnosis and create a treatment plan tailored to your needs.

6. Be aware of risk factors: Certain risk factors, such as a family history of mental illness, traumatic experiences, or chronic stress, can increase the likelihood of developing a mental health issue. If you are aware of these risk factors, you can take steps to reduce their impact or seek professional help before symptoms develop.

7. Know when to seek emergency help: If you or a loved one is experiencing severe symptoms, such as suicidal thoughts, hallucinations, or delusions, it's important to seek emergency help immediately. Call your local emergency services or go to the nearest emergency room.

Overall, identifying signs and symptoms of mental health issues can be challenging, but it's an important step in early intervention and treatment. By paying attention to changes in mood, behavior, and physical symptoms, seeking professional help, and being aware of risk factors, you can take steps to improve your mental health and well-being.

Chapter 4: Understanding Medical Reports and Test Results

Interpreting medical reports and lab test results

Interpreting medical reports and lab test results can be a daunting task, especially for those who are unfamiliar with medical terminology and concepts. However, it is an essential skill to have in order to fully understand one's health status and make informed decisions regarding their healthcare. In this chapter, we will discuss the basics of interpreting medical reports and lab test results.

Medical Reports

Medical reports are documents generated by healthcare professionals that contain information about a patient's health status, including medical history, physical examination findings, laboratory test results, and imaging studies. Medical reports are important because they provide a snapshot of a patient's health status at a specific point in time. Interpreting medical reports requires an understanding of medical terminology and the ability to identify abnormal findings.

There are several components of a medical report, including the following:

1. Patient information: This includes the patient's name, age, sex, and other identifying information.

2. Medical history: This includes information about the patient's past medical conditions, surgeries, allergies, and medications.

3. Physical examination findings: This includes information about the patient's current symptoms, vital signs, and any abnormal findings on physical examination.

4. Laboratory test results: This includes the results of blood tests, urine tests, and other diagnostic tests that can provide information about a patient's health status.

Interpreting Laboratory Test Results

Laboratory tests are an important tool for healthcare professionals in diagnosing and monitoring various medical conditions. Interpreting laboratory test results requires an understanding of what each test measures and what the normal ranges for each test are. It is important to note that normal ranges may vary depending on the laboratory that performs the test.

The following are some common laboratory tests and what they measure:

1. Complete blood count (CBC): This measures the levels of red blood cells, white blood cells, and platelets in the blood. Abnormalities in the CBC can indicate various medical conditions, such as anemia or infection.

2. Blood chemistry panel: This measures the levels of various substances in the blood, such as glucose, electrolytes, and liver enzymes. Abnormalities in the blood chemistry panel can indicate various medical conditions, such as diabetes or liver disease.

3. Urinalysis: This measures the contents of urine, including protein, glucose, and other substances. Abnormalities in the urinalysis can indicate various medical conditions, such as kidney disease or urinary tract infections.

4. Imaging studies: This includes X-rays, CT scans, and MRI scans, which provide images of the body's internal structures. Abnormalities in imaging studies can indicate various medical conditions, such as bone fractures or tumors.

It is important to note that laboratory test results should always be interpreted in the context of a patient's medical history and physical examination findings. Abnormal laboratory test results may indicate the need for further testing or evaluation by a healthcare professional.

Conclusion

Interpreting medical reports and lab test results can be challenging, but it is an essential skill for anyone who wants to fully understand their health status. By understanding the basics of medical terminology and the normal ranges for various laboratory tests, patients can be more informed about their health and better equipped to make decisions about their healthcare. It is important to remember that laboratory test results should always be interpreted in the context of a patient's medical history and physical examination findings, and any abnormalities should be further evaluated by a healthcare professional.

How to communicate effectively with healthcare providers

Communicating effectively with healthcare providers is an important aspect of maintaining good health. It is essential to develop a positive and effective relationship with healthcare providers, which involves effective communication skills. In this chapter, we will discuss various aspects of communication with healthcare providers, including how to communicate effectively, how to prepare for appointments, and how to ask questions to ensure that you understand your medical reports and test results.

Preparing for Appointments

Preparing for appointments with healthcare providers is essential for effective communication. Patients should have a clear idea of their medical history, including any relevant health information and medical reports. Patients should prepare a list of questions to ask their healthcare providers, including questions about their medical reports and test results.

It is also essential to bring a list of medications, including over-the-counter drugs and supplements, to the appointment. Patients should inform their healthcare providers of any allergies or adverse reactions they may have experienced in the past. Providing healthcare providers with detailed information about your medical history can help them provide accurate diagnoses and treatment plans.

Communicating Effectively

Effective communication with healthcare providers involves more than just providing accurate medical history and a list of questions. It is essential to communicate clearly and confidently to ensure that healthcare providers understand your concerns and medical conditions.

Patients should describe their symptoms clearly, using specific terms such as "sharp" or "dull" pain. It is also important to describe the severity and duration of symptoms, as well as any patterns or triggers. Patients should also inform their healthcare providers of any lifestyle changes, such as changes in diet, exercise, or sleep habits.

Asking Questions

Asking questions is an important aspect of effective communication with healthcare providers. Patients should ask questions to ensure that they understand their medical reports and test results. Patients should also ask questions to understand their diagnoses and treatment plans, including potential side effects and medication interactions.

Patients should not be afraid to ask questions or express their concerns. It is essential to develop a partnership with healthcare providers based on trust and open communication. Patients should be encouraged to seek clarification if they do not understand medical terminology or jargon.

Conclusion

Effective communication with healthcare providers is an essential aspect of maintaining good health. Patients should prepare for appointments, communicate clearly, and ask questions to ensure that they understand their medical reports and test results. Developing a positive and effective relationship with healthcare providers can help patients receive accurate diagnoses and effective treatment plans. It is essential to take an active role in your healthcare by communicating effectively with your healthcare providers.

Understanding medical jargon

Medical jargon can be difficult to understand, but it is essential to decipher it in order to understand your medical reports and test results accurately. Medical jargon is a specialized vocabulary used by healthcare professionals, and it can include complex medical terms and acronyms.

Here are some tips to help you better understand medical jargon:

1. Ask your healthcare provider to explain terms: If you do not understand a term or acronym used in your medical report or test result, do not hesitate to ask your healthcare provider to explain it. They will be happy to provide you with an explanation that you can understand.

2. Use online resources: There are several online resources available that can help you understand medical jargon. Websites such as MedlinePlus, Mayo Clinic, and WebMD provide an extensive list of medical terms and their definitions.

3. Break down the word: Medical terms can often be broken down into smaller parts, which can help you understand their meaning. For example, the medical term "cardiomyopathy" can be broken down into "cardio" meaning heart, "myo" meaning muscle, and "pathy" meaning

disease. Therefore, cardiomyopathy refers to a disease of the heart muscle.

4. Context: Understanding the context in which a medical term is used can help you better understand its meaning. For example, if you see the term "ECG" in your medical report, it may be referring to an electrocardiogram, which is a test that measures the electrical activity of the heart.

5. Learn common medical terms: Learning common medical terms can help you better understand medical jargon. Some common medical terms include:

- Diagnosis: Identifying a disease or condition based on symptoms, medical history, and test results.

- Prognosis: Predicting the outcome of a disease or condition.

- Treatment: A plan of action designed to improve a patient's health.

- Symptom: A sign of a disease or condition that a patient experiences.

- Diagnosis code: A code used by healthcare providers to identify a patient's diagnosis for billing and insurance purposes.

6. Be patient: Understanding medical jargon takes time and patience. Do not be discouraged if you do not

understand everything at first. Keep asking questions and learning new terms, and you will eventually build a strong foundation of medical knowledge.

In conclusion, understanding medical jargon is crucial for comprehending medical reports and test results accurately. By asking questions, using online resources, breaking down words, understanding the context, learning common medical terms, and being patient, you can improve your understanding of medical jargon and better communicate with your healthcare provider.

Chapter 5: Special Considerations for Different Age Groups

Age-appropriate health screenings

As we age, our bodies undergo various changes, which make us more susceptible to certain health conditions. Therefore, it's important to get age-appropriate health screenings to detect and prevent any potential health problems early on. In this chapter, we'll discuss the age-appropriate health screenings that are recommended for different age groups.

1. Children and Adolescents Children and adolescents should receive regular check-ups and screenings to monitor their growth and development, as well as to identify any health problems that may require treatment. Some of the age-appropriate health screenings for this age group include:

- Physical exams: Children should receive regular physical exams to check their growth and development, as well as to monitor their weight and height.

- Vision and hearing screenings: Vision and hearing problems can affect a child's ability to learn and develop. Regular screenings can help detect any issues early on.

- Dental exams: Regular dental check-ups are essential for maintaining good oral health and preventing dental problems.

- Immunizations: Children should receive vaccines to protect them against various diseases, such as measles, mumps, rubella, and chickenpox.

2. Young Adults Young adults should continue to receive regular check-ups and screenings to monitor their overall health and detect any potential health problems. Some of the age-appropriate health screenings for this age group include:

- Blood pressure screening: High blood pressure can increase the risk of heart disease and stroke. Regular screenings can help detect any issues early on.

- Cholesterol screening: High cholesterol levels can increase the risk of heart disease. Regular screenings can help identify any issues and allow for early intervention.

- Skin exams: Young adults should receive regular skin exams to detect any potential skin cancer.

- STD testing: Sexually transmitted diseases are common among young adults. Regular testing can help detect any issues early on.

3. Middle-aged Adults Middle-aged adults should continue to receive regular check-ups and screenings to monitor their overall health and detect any potential health problems. Some of the age-appropriate health screenings for this age group include:

- Colon cancer screening: Colon cancer is a common type of cancer among middle-aged adults. Regular screenings can help detect any potential issues early on.

- Mammography: Women should receive regular mammograms to screen for breast cancer.

- Bone density screening: Women should receive regular bone density screenings to detect any potential issues with bone health.

- Prostate cancer screening: Men should receive regular prostate cancer screenings to detect any potential issues early on.

4. Older Adults Older adults should continue to receive regular check-ups and screenings to monitor their overall health and detect any potential health problems. Some of the age-appropriate health screenings for this age group include:

- Eye exams: Older adults are at a higher risk of developing eye problems, such as cataracts and glaucoma. Regular eye exams can help detect any issues early on.

- Hearing exams: Older adults are at a higher risk of developing hearing problems. Regular hearing exams can help detect any issues early on.

- Osteoporosis screening: Older adults are at a higher risk of developing osteoporosis. Regular screenings can help detect any potential issues with bone health.

- Memory screenings: Older adults are at a higher risk of developing memory problems, such as dementia. Regular memory screenings can help detect any issues early on.

In conclusion, age-appropriate health screenings are essential for maintaining good health and preventing potential health problems. By getting regular check-ups and screenings, you can stay on top of your health and detect any issues early on, allowing for early intervention and treatment.

Understanding common health risks for different age groups

As people age, they become more vulnerable to certain health risks. The body undergoes various changes, and the risk of developing certain conditions increases. Being aware of these risks can help individuals take steps to prevent or manage them. Below are some common health risks associated with different age groups.

Children and adolescents During childhood and adolescence, the body undergoes significant physical and emotional changes. This can make children and teenagers more vulnerable to certain health risks, including:

1. Childhood obesity: Childhood obesity has become a major health concern in recent years. Children who are overweight or obese are at increased risk of developing a range of health problems, including type 2 diabetes, high blood pressure, and heart disease. Encouraging children to eat a healthy diet and get regular exercise can help reduce their risk of obesity.

2. Substance abuse: Substance abuse is a major problem among teenagers. It can lead to a range of physical and mental health problems, as well as legal problems. Parents and caregivers can help reduce the risk of substance

abuse by talking to their children about the dangers of drugs and alcohol and monitoring their behavior.

3. Mental health problems: Mental health problems are common among children and teenagers. These can include anxiety, depression, and behavioral disorders. It's important for parents and caregivers to be aware of the signs of these conditions and seek help if necessary.

Adults As people enter adulthood, their risk of developing certain health problems increases. Some common health risks for adults include:

1. Cardiovascular disease: Cardiovascular disease is the leading cause of death among adults in many countries. Risk factors for cardiovascular disease include smoking, high blood pressure, high cholesterol, and diabetes. Eating a healthy diet, getting regular exercise, and avoiding tobacco can help reduce the risk of cardiovascular disease.

2. Cancer: The risk of developing cancer increases with age. Some of the most common types of cancer in adults include lung cancer, breast cancer, and prostate cancer. Regular cancer screenings can help detect cancer early, when it's most treatable.

3. Mental health problems: Mental health problems are not limited to children and teenagers. Adults can also experience anxiety, depression, and other mental health

conditions. Seeking help from a mental health professional can be beneficial.

Older adults As people age into their senior years, they become more vulnerable to certain health problems. Some common health risks for older adults include:

1. Falls: Falls are a major health concern for older adults. They can lead to serious injuries, including broken bones and head injuries. Older adults can reduce their risk of falls by staying physically active, getting regular vision check-ups, and making modifications to their home environment.

2. Dementia: Dementia is a group of conditions that affect memory, thinking, and behavior. It becomes more common with age. There are several types of dementia, including Alzheimer's disease. There is no cure for dementia, but early diagnosis and treatment can help slow the progression of the disease.

3. Chronic diseases: Older adults are at increased risk of developing chronic diseases, such as arthritis, diabetes, and heart disease. These conditions can have a significant impact on quality of life. Managing these conditions with the help of a healthcare provider can help reduce the risk of complications.

Conclusion Being aware of common health risks associated with different age groups is an important step in maintaining good health. By understanding these risks, individuals can take steps to prevent or manage them. It's also important to seek regular medical check-ups and screenings to detect any health problems early.

Preventive care for children, adults, and seniors

Preventive care is important for people of all ages, as it can help to identify health problems early on, when they are most treatable. However, the specific preventive care needs of children, adults, and seniors can vary significantly due to differences in their health risks and developmental stages. In this section, we will discuss preventive care recommendations for each age group, including children, adults, and seniors.

Preventive Care for Children

Preventive care for children includes a range of screenings, vaccinations, and health assessments that are critical to their overall health and development. Some important components of preventive care for children include:

1. Vaccinations: Childhood vaccinations are a critical component of preventive care. Vaccinations help to protect children from serious illnesses, such as measles, mumps, rubella, and polio. The Centers for Disease Control and Prevention (CDC) recommends a schedule of vaccinations for children from birth through age 18.

2. Well-child visits: Well-child visits are an important opportunity for healthcare providers to assess a child's

growth and development, as well as to provide guidance on nutrition, safety, and other important health issues.

3. Vision and hearing screenings: Regular vision and hearing screenings can help to identify problems early on and ensure that children receive the necessary treatment.

4. Dental check-ups: Regular dental check-ups can help to prevent tooth decay and gum disease, as well as identify any potential dental problems early on.

5. Screenings for developmental delays: Early screenings for developmental delays can help to identify problems early on, when they are most treatable. Screenings may include assessments of a child's cognitive, social, and emotional development.

Preventive Care for Adults

Preventive care for adults includes a range of screenings, vaccinations, and health assessments that are critical to maintaining good health and preventing disease. Some important components of preventive care for adults include:

1. Vaccinations: Like children, adults also need to stay up to date on vaccinations to protect against serious illnesses, such as influenza, pneumococcal disease, and shingles.

2. Annual physical exams: Annual physical exams can help to identify potential health problems early on, as well as provide an opportunity for healthcare providers to discuss lifestyle factors that may impact health.

3. Cancer screenings: Cancer screenings, such as mammograms and colonoscopies, can help to identify cancer early on, when it is most treatable.

4. Blood pressure and cholesterol checks: Regular checks of blood pressure and cholesterol levels can help to identify potential risk factors for heart disease and stroke.

5. Diabetes screenings: Diabetes is a common chronic disease that can be managed effectively with early detection and treatment. Regular diabetes screenings can help to identify the disease early on, when it is most treatable.

Preventive Care for Seniors

As people age, their risk for certain health problems, such as chronic diseases and falls, increases. Preventive care for seniors includes a range of screenings, vaccinations, and health assessments that are critical to maintaining good health and preventing disease. Some important components of preventive care for seniors include:

1. Vaccinations: Seniors need to stay up to date on vaccinations, particularly for flu and pneumonia, to protect against serious illnesses.

2. Annual physical exams: Annual physical exams can help to identify potential health problems early on, as well as provide an opportunity for healthcare providers to discuss lifestyle factors that may impact health.

3. Cancer screenings: Cancer screenings, such as mammograms and colonoscopies, can help to identify cancer early on, when it is most treatable.

4. Bone density screenings: Bone density screenings can help to identify osteoporosis, a common condition in seniors that increases the risk of fractures.

5. Fall risk assessments: Falls are a common problem in seniors and can result in serious injuries.

Chapter 6: Overcoming Barriers to Regular Check-Ups

Financial and insurance barriers to care

Access to healthcare can be limited by various factors, including financial and insurance barriers. Even individuals who understand the importance of preventive care may face challenges when it comes to receiving regular check-ups. Addressing financial and insurance barriers is an essential step towards promoting preventive care and ensuring that all individuals have access to essential health services. In this section, we will explore some of the financial and insurance barriers that can prevent individuals from receiving regular check-ups and discuss potential solutions to overcome these barriers.

1. Cost of healthcare One of the primary financial barriers to preventive care is the cost of healthcare. Many individuals are unable to afford the high costs associated with routine check-ups, which can include the cost of doctor visits, lab tests, and imaging studies. Without insurance coverage, the out-of-pocket costs of healthcare can be prohibitively expensive, even for basic services.

2. Lack of insurance coverage Another significant barrier to preventive care is the lack of insurance coverage. Without insurance, individuals may be unable to afford

regular check-ups, diagnostic tests, and other essential health services. Even individuals who have insurance may face limitations on coverage or high deductibles and co-pays, which can discourage them from seeking care.

3. Limited access to care In addition to financial barriers, many individuals face limited access to care due to their geographic location or other factors. Individuals who live in rural or remote areas may struggle to find healthcare providers, while those who live in low-income or underserved areas may have difficulty accessing medical facilities or services. Language barriers and cultural differences can also create obstacles to care, making it challenging for some individuals to receive preventive services.

4. Fear and mistrust of the healthcare system Finally, fear and mistrust of the healthcare system can also prevent individuals from seeking preventive care. Some individuals may have had negative experiences with healthcare providers in the past, while others may be hesitant to undergo screening tests or receive medical treatment due to cultural or religious beliefs.

Overcoming Financial and Insurance Barriers to Preventive Care

1. Health insurance coverage One of the most effective ways to overcome financial barriers to preventive care is to ensure that all individuals have access to health insurance coverage. Under the Affordable Care Act (ACA), most Americans are required to have health insurance or face a penalty. The ACA also provides subsidies to help individuals and families afford health insurance premiums, making coverage more accessible for low-income individuals.

2. Employer-sponsored health insurance Many employers offer health insurance as part of their benefits package. This can be an affordable way for individuals to obtain health insurance coverage, especially if their employer subsidizes the cost of premiums. Employers may also offer flexible spending accounts or health savings accounts, which can help employees save money on healthcare costs.

3. Government-funded health programs For individuals who are uninsured or underinsured, government-funded health programs may be available. Medicaid provides health coverage to low-income individuals and families, while Medicare provides coverage for individuals aged 65 and older. The Children's Health Insurance Program (CHIP) provides coverage to children in low-income families who do not qualify for Medicaid.

4. Community health clinics Community health clinics are another resource for individuals who face financial barriers to preventive care. These clinics provide low-cost or free medical services to individuals who cannot afford to pay for care. Some community health clinics offer sliding scale fees, which are based on income, to make care more affordable for low-income individuals.

5. Telehealth services Telehealth services can also help overcome financial and insurance barriers to preventive care. Telehealth allows patients to connect with healthcare providers remotely, using video conferencing or other technology. This can be a cost-effective way to receive medical advice, screening tests, and other essential health services without having to travel to a medical facility.

In conclusion, financial and insurance barriers can prevent individuals from receiving regular check-ups and preventive care, leading to undiagnosed and untreated health conditions that can ultimately result in more serious and costly health problems. However, there are various resources and strategies available to help overcome these barriers and ensure access to necessary medical care. One such resource is Medicaid, a joint federal and state program that provides healthcare coverage to eligible low-income individuals and families. Medicaid covers many preventive services, including regular check-ups, cancer screenings, and vaccinations, at little to no cost for enrollees. Other strategies for overcoming financial barriers to care include seeking out community health clinics, negotiating payment plans with healthcare providers, and utilizing healthcare savings accounts. Additionally, advocacy efforts to expand access to healthcare for all individuals, regardless of income or insurance status, can help address systemic barriers to preventive care.

Overcoming fear and anxiety about medical exams

Medical exams can evoke fear and anxiety in many individuals, leading them to avoid seeking regular check-ups altogether. This fear can stem from various sources, such as a fear of needles or medical procedures, fear of receiving a negative diagnosis, or a lack of trust in healthcare providers. However, regular check-ups are crucial for maintaining good health, preventing disease, and identifying potential health issues early on. Here are some strategies for overcoming fear and anxiety about medical exams:

1. Educate yourself about the exam: Knowing what to expect during a medical exam can help alleviate fear and anxiety. You can ask your healthcare provider about the exam process and any potential discomfort that may occur. Additionally, you can research the exam online to learn more about it and prepare yourself mentally.

2. Practice relaxation techniques: Deep breathing, meditation, and visualization exercises can help you relax before and during a medical exam. These techniques can help calm your nerves and reduce anxiety.

3. Seek support from a trusted individual: Having someone you trust, such as a family member or friend, accompany you to the exam can provide emotional support and reassurance.

4. Communicate your fears with your healthcare provider: It's important to communicate any fears or concerns you may have with your healthcare provider. They can offer support, guidance, and may even be able to provide medication or other interventions to help you relax.

5. Consider therapy: If your fear and anxiety about medical exams are severe and impacting your quality of life, you may want to consider therapy. A therapist can help you work through your fears and develop coping strategies to manage them.

Remember, regular check-ups are essential for maintaining good health and identifying potential health issues early on. Overcoming fear and anxiety about medical exams is a critical step towards prioritizing your health and well-being.

The role of patient education in preventive care

Patient education plays a critical role in preventive care. By educating patients about the importance of regular check-ups and screenings, as well as healthy lifestyle habits, they can become active participants in their own health care. When patients have a good understanding of their health and the importance of preventive care, they are more likely to schedule regular check-ups and screenings, as well as take steps to maintain their health.

One of the most effective ways to educate patients about preventive care is through patient education materials. These materials can include brochures, handouts, and online resources that provide information on a variety of topics related to preventive care, including:

1. The importance of regular check-ups: Patients need to understand the importance of regular check-ups and the role they play in maintaining good health. Educating patients about the benefits of preventive care can motivate them to schedule regular appointments and participate in screenings.

2. Health screenings: Patients need to know what screenings are recommended for their age group and how often they should receive them. Patient education materials can provide this information and help patients understand the significance of these tests.

3. Healthy lifestyle habits: Patient education materials can also provide information on healthy lifestyle habits that can help prevent disease, such as exercise, healthy eating, and stress management.

4. Understanding medical terminology: Medical terminology can be confusing and overwhelming for patients. Patient education materials can help patients understand medical terms and concepts so they can better understand their health care providers and their own health.

5. Managing chronic conditions: For patients with chronic conditions, patient education materials can provide information on how to manage their condition and prevent complications.

Patient education materials can be distributed in a variety of ways, including in-office handouts, online resources, and social media. Health care providers can also use patient education materials during appointments to discuss preventive care with their patients and answer any questions they may have.

In addition to patient education materials, health care providers can also provide education through one-on-one counseling sessions. These sessions allow providers to discuss preventive care and healthy lifestyle habits with patients in more detail and address any specific concerns or questions patients may have.

By providing patient education on preventive care, health care providers can help patients become more engaged in their own health care and reduce the barriers that may prevent them from receiving regular check-ups and screenings. With the right knowledge and resources, patients can take charge of their health and make informed decisions about their health care.

Conclusion"
The Importance of Taking Action

In conclusion, regular medical check-ups are essential for maintaining good health and preventing disease. Taking action to prioritize preventive care can help individuals identify potential health issues early on and improve overall health outcomes. While there may be barriers to accessing regular check-ups, such as financial and insurance challenges, fear and anxiety, or lack of patient education, there are strategies for overcoming these barriers and prioritizing preventive care.

One important way to take action is to make regular check-ups a priority in one's life. This can involve scheduling appointments well in advance, setting reminders, and making sure to attend appointments even when feeling healthy. Another way to take action is to educate oneself about preventive care and the different types of exams and screenings that are recommended based on age and health history. This can help individuals feel more confident and prepared when attending appointments and speaking with healthcare providers.

Another important step in taking action is to advocate for oneself when it comes to accessing care. This may involve researching and selecting insurance plans that provide coverage for preventive care, or working with healthcare providers to find affordable options for services. In some cases, it may also be helpful to reach out to community organizations or government programs that can provide assistance with healthcare costs.

Overall, taking action to prioritize preventive care and overcome barriers to accessing regular check-ups is essential for promoting optimal health and well-being. By staying informed and proactive about one's health, individuals can ensure they receive the care they need to stay healthy and prevent disease.

Looking Towards the Future

As we move forward, it is important to recognize that healthcare and preventive care are constantly evolving. New research and technology allow for improved methods of detection and treatment, and it is important to stay informed and up-to-date on these advancements.

One area of great potential is in the field of personalized medicine. This approach takes into account an individual's unique genetic makeup, lifestyle factors, and other personal characteristics to develop personalized prevention and treatment plans. This could lead to more effective and targeted preventive care, reducing the overall burden of disease.

Another area of focus is on increasing access to preventive care, particularly for underserved populations. This may involve expanding insurance coverage, increasing funding for community health clinics, and improving healthcare infrastructure in rural areas.

It is also important to continue to emphasize the importance of preventive care and regular check-ups, both for individuals and for society as a whole. This can be achieved through public health campaigns, education, and policy initiatives that prioritize preventive care and make it more accessible to all.

By taking action now to prioritize preventive care and overcome barriers to regular check-ups, we can improve health outcomes and reduce the burden of disease for ourselves and future generations. It is up to all of us to make our health a priority and to work towards a healthier future for all.

THE END

Potential References

Introduction:

- World Health Organization. (2020). Universal Health Coverage. Retrieved from https://www.who.int/healthsystems/universal_health_coverage/en/

Chapter 1: The Basics of Regular Medical Check-Ups:

- American Heart Association. (2021). Know Your Numbers: Blood Pressure. Retrieved from https://www.heart.org/en/health-topics/high-blood-pressure/know-your-numbers

- American Cancer Society. (2022). Cancer Screening Guidelines. Retrieved from https://www.cancer.org/healthy/find-cancer-early/cancer-screening-guidelines.html

Chapter 2: Physical Exams and Screening Tests:

- U.S. Preventive Services Task Force. (2021). Screening for High Blood Pressure in Adults: U.S. Preventive Services Task Force Recommendation Statement. JAMA, 325(19), 1972-1980.

- American Heart Association. (2021). Understanding Cholesterol. Retrieved from https://www.heart.org/en/health-topics/cholesterol

Chapter 3: Mental Health Screenings:

- National Alliance on Mental Illness. (2021). Mental Health Conditions. Retrieved from https://www.nami.org/About-Mental-Illness/Mental-Health-Conditions
- Substance Abuse and Mental Health Services Administration. (2016). The Role of Behavioral Health in Addressing the Social Determinants of Health. Retrieved from https://store.samhsa.gov/product/The-Role-of-Behavioral-Health-in-Addressing-the-Social-Determinants-of-Health/SMA16-4956

Chapter 4: Understanding Medical Reports and Test Results:
- American Medical Association. (2022). How to Read Your Medical Bills. Retrieved from https://www.ama-assn.org/practice-management/billing-insurance/how-read-your-medical-bills
- National Cancer Institute. (2021). Understanding Your Pathology Report. Retrieved from https://www.cancer.gov/about-cancer/diagnosis-staging/understanding-pathology-report

Chapter 5: Special Considerations for Different Age Groups:
- Centers for Disease Control and Prevention. (2021). Recommended Child and Adolescent Immunization Schedule for ages 18 years or younger, United States, 2021. Retrieved from

https://www.cdc.gov/vaccines/schedules/hcp/imz/child-adolescent.html

- U.S. Department of Health and Human Services. (2021). Health Screenings for Women: MedlinePlus Medical Encyclopedia. Retrieved from https://medlineplus.gov/ency/article/007467.htm

Chapter 6: Overcoming Barriers to Regular Check-Ups:

- American College of Physicians. (2017). Addressing Social Determinants to Improve Patient Care and Promote Health Equity: An American College of Physicians Position Paper. Annals of Internal Medicine, 168(8), 577-578.

- Centers for Medicare & Medicaid Services. (2021). Coverage for Overcoming Barriers to Care. Retrieved from https://www.cms.gov/CCIIO/Programs-and-Initiatives/Other-Insurance-Protections/Overcoming-Barriers-to-Care

Conclusion

- World Health Organization. (2021). Strengthening integrated people-centred health services: Report of the Regional Director. Retrieved from https://apps.who.int/iris/handle/10665/340474

- American Medical Association. (2022). What is Health Equity? Retrieved from https://www.ama-assn.org/delivering-care/health-equity

www.ingramcontent.com/pod-product-compliance
Lightning Source LLC
LaVergne TN
LVHW012127070526
838202LV00056B/5898